If your Mother
never told you

If your Mother never told you

Crystal Ferguson

To order additional copies of this book, contact:
Xlibris
1-888-795-4274
www.Xlibris.com
Orders@Xlibris.com
76855

Contents

Introduction

THIS book was created in the hopes of informing and diverting my young sisters who are reiterating a cycle of disappointments as well as hardships. My direction is to build an environment that creates educated and powerful young sisters who will accomplish a completed education, which in return will definitely allow them the chance at a successful career. My sole purpose is to produce as well as display every opportunity that's available to our fortunate sisters and allow that same opportunity to present itself to our unfortunate sisters. In addition, my focus is to build each and every young sister's self-esteem level and guide them through a variety of everyday issues as well as solutions that young women face in today's society.

Prayer

May God protect each young sister reading these words. May he guide you into a light of complete understanding and allow you the chance to start life on the right foot as opposed to starting late in life faced with difficult challenges. I pray he send down the angels to cover your body from any forms of harm and clear your vision so that you can choose the correct road to travel. I pray that God bless you and place you in a safe environment for you and your child. I pray God heals your heart and removes any forms of hatred and instead fills your heart with love and forgiveness. I pray he carries you when you are weak and unable to walk. I pray he supplies your every need and blesses you with treasures that no man can take away. Amen.

Bathtub/Shower

THIS day and age is completely different from three and four generations ago. I can remember my grandmother preparing the bathtub and coming in the bathroom to wash me up. My grandmother would often say "You can't clean yourself properly, you're too young."

What I often remember about my grandmother was during the time she was washing me, she would explain what she was doing and why she was doing it. She would grab my arms and say "I know you're not used to being washed up, but in this house, we go to bed clean and fresh." The funny thing is my cousins that I went to visit already knew she was going to do this because she washes all the grandkids.

The difference between my grandmother and my mother was my grandmother washed us, and my mother told us how to wash. My mother would say things like "clean in them ears" and "wash in between them cracks." Life is so funny, and it just repeats itself because what they instilled in me will follow me for a lifetime.

The more I matured, the more I understood that taking care of the body is very important. I went from rushing in the bathtub to sitting, relaxing, and soaking in the bathtub. Some of my friends preferred a shower as opposed to a bath, but what I realized was a bath cleanses inside the woman's private area when soaking in the tub.

When I sit in the tub, I receive a better feel than I do when taking a shower. Some women feel like sitting in the bathtub keeps the dirt on you and taking a shower cleanses the dirt off your body and sends it straight down the drain. Whatever a woman chooses to do, I suggest she use two washcloths, one for her private area and the other for her face, because cleaning the private area and cleaning the face with the same washcloth is transferring germs.

Underarm Hair/Hair on the Legs

I must admit the hair under my arms as well as on my legs never affected me until I wore a sleeveless dress one day and I raised my arms, and all I could see was clunks of deodorant under my armpits. I was so embarrassed. My mother would often tell me to shave my armpits, but I never listened to what she was saying. When I reached the stages of an adult, I began to understand the importance of removing the hair in my armpits and on my legs. I would hear some of my girlfriends say the best solution to remove hair is to visit a spa that specializes in removal of the unwanted hair.

This topic is kind of complicated because some young sisters are not concerned about the hair on their legs and their armpits, but then on the other hand, you have sisters who remove the hair often.

The only problem I have with the hair on my legs is when the summertime approaches and the weather is extremely warm. I usually shave the unwanted hair in the shower with a shaving razor. Below I mentioned a few steps to removing unwanted hair on the legs and the armpits.

- There are spas that specialize in removing unwanted hair by waxing the armpits.
- There are products you can purchase to remove unwanted hair.
- There are shaving clippers you can purchase to remove the hair yourself.

Clothing that Should Not Be Worn Out of the Home

1 – US growing woman should never ever come outside the home with a comb stuck to the back of our heads. It sends a message that we are not concerned about our appearance. Our hair should be combed and neatly cropped before the thought of leaving your homes even occurs. If your hair is not done, then I recommend a very nice ponytail pulled to the back of your head.

2 – Scarves

If a woman chooses to wear scarves on her head, then she should purchase designer scarves and wear the scarves in a stylish way. The scarf can be tied in a bun to the back of the head, it can be wrapped around the head in a circular motion, or it can be worn in a bun turned to the side of your head. Ladies, it's how you are wearing your scarves that are attracting the negative stares that you receive when you are on the train, at the supermarket, or just riding the bus. Your appearance says who you are and how you take care of yourself.

3 – Slippers

They should not be worn outside the home; they are not shoes, and they should not be worn to the corner store. In addition, slippers should not be worn on the job! When I wear heels, I carry a pair of flats or a pair of loafers in my bag so that I can change if my feet start to bother me. A young woman should always look presentable. When you go to the store to purchase slippers, you ask for house slippers; the name is telling you what they should be used for. Throughout my entire life, I have heard the words chicken heads or hood rats. These are terms that are used for women who do not have a good appearance. The older I become, I realize that our young sisters should not be called these names and instead they should be taught the correct way so that they can be called a queen and a princess.

When young women wear slippers outside the home, they pick up all the germs that are on the sidewalks and in the streets, and they track these same germs back inside of their home. If a person's home is complete with carpets, these germs are transferred to the rugs that are on the floor in your home. Slippers are made to be worn in the home.

Pajamas

There should be no reasons as well as excuses as to why pajamas are worn as clothing outside of the home. For a number of years, I have witnessed young women completely comfortable with getting out of their beds and walking straight to the corner store. What is even more disturbing is the fact that this trend is being passed down from generation to generation. When I began to notice young sisters outside dressed in their pajamas, I started thinking of a way to cease and create a better direction for our sisters.

Before a plan is created, we need to first find out the reason for this action. I asked a couple of young women why do they come outside dressed in their pajamas? Below you will see their responses.

- One sister said it is quicker to run to the store.
- Another sister said this is what she wears until she gets dressed for the day.

When asking this question, you also receive responses like "it's none of your business." Besides the fact that this is a trend, I truly believe its existence is so strong because our young women lack self-esteem. When a young woman contains self-esteem, this type of action would never exist.

Clothing that Should Be Worn on an Interview

WHEN a young woman is going on an interview, there are a variety of things she needs to know. The interviewer is going to watch the person she or he is interviewing. The first thing a young woman needs to do is relax and answer each question with clarity. It is always an excellent thing to have an extensive vocabulary and the ability to complete full sentences. Whenever a young woman goes on an interview, she should always arrive on time. Every woman needs to achieve a business-look attire. A nice black or dark blue suit, a nice pair of pumps, and a nice set of pearls is the look that would complete a great interview. If a woman has very long hair, a nice neat bun is suitable for the interview. I think it's best not to overdress your look.

Items We Do Not Wear on an Interview

Every young sister needs to understand that her appearance is very important when she goes on an interview. Yes, it's true that once you're on an interview, you will be asked a variety of questions about your past job titles, what you specialized in, and your educational background. What people do not know is your etiquette and appearance will be taken into consideration also. Make sure you're always on time or before the time they expect you to arrive but never ever do you arrive late to an interview. If you do show up late to an interview, the company will label you as being an unreliable individual.

The majority of the time the person who is conducting the interview will know almost instantly if you are the person that the company is looking for.

Here are some items we should never ever wear on an interview:

1. Jeans
2. Spandex
3. Big hoop earrings
4. Sweat suits
5. Tight clothing
6. A large amount of bracelets
7. Strong-smelling perfume
8. Colorful hairstreaks
9. Bright nail polish
10. Colorful clothing
11. See-through tops
12. Sneakers

Each item that I just mentioned should not be worn on an interview. When you are on an interview, you want to be taken very seriously and you do not want to distract the person who is interviewing you. Most of the garments I mentioned above I usually wear on the weekend, and some of the items I refuse to wear. Take your time when you are trying to find the correct outfit to wear on this interview, and remember you only have one chance to impress the person who is interviewing you.

Shirts

OKAY, it's just a shirt; or is it? Sisters, when you wake up in the morning and you decide what you are going to wear for that day, just keep in mind that a respectable young woman does not reveal the size of her breast. Each time we purchase a shirt, we must be aware of the type of shirt we purchase. If we buy a shirt that is sheer, then we should consider a T-shirt under our shirt.

If we purchase a jean shirt, then we do not need to wear a T-shirt under this shirt. What I see young women do is revealing too much of their breasts. There's nothing wrong with wearing sheer shirts, but just be careful and always wear something under the shirt. When you wear revealing shirts, you will receive unwanted and disrespectful attention.

Braids

MY beautiful young sisters, I have a few words to say about this topic. Let me first start by saying if braids are what you choose to wear, make sure the braids are clean and neat. Let me give you a few pointers. When you have braids in your hair, you can still wash the braids. After you wash the braids, dry the braids and apply hair spray for a nice shine. In addition, if your funds are low and you cannot afford to get your braids redone, take each braid and redo it yourself. As a young woman, do not ever use lack of funds to be the reason why you do not keep your hair looking nice. Be sure to brush your braids to remove any forms of lint in your hair. Another way to keep your braids neat is to wear a silk scarf to bed at night.

Fingernails

SISTERS, sisters, sisters. Each sister must understand the importance of pretty and clean fingernails. We are women, and our nails must be clean at all times. Let me first tell you that you do not need to wear nail tips to keep your nails looking nice. If you choose to wear nail polish, make sure the polish you wear is not chipped because it sends a message to people that you're not a neat person. Let me also inform you that you do not have to go to the nail salon to get your nails done because the same products they have in the nail salon you can purchase at the hair store. Take the time out and file your nails evenly. You can also apply nail oil to remove the dry skin around your cuticles. The most important thing about nails is to keep them clean at all times.

Toenails

WHEN the summertime arrives and we wear our sandals, our feet should be clean and our toenails nicely painted. Anytime women's feet are being shown, there should always be pure beauty visible. Whenever I get out of the shower, I use a large amount of Vaseline. I rub it all over my feet, and then I put the heaviest socks on. When my toenails are painted, I do not always go to the nail salon; most of the time I paint my own nails. I soak my feet in a bucket of water, I pour a few drops of bleach in the water, I soak for a while, dry my feet, and then I polish my toenails. The same products that they have in the nail salon you can buy and keep them in your home.

Douche

THIS is a topic I must speak in detail about! One day a young woman who often confides in me approached me and asked me what a douche was. I was completely shocked. My response to her question was a douche is used to clean the vagina after sex and after your menstrual cycle (period) is over.

I mentioned to her that another way I cleanse the vagina when I want a fresh feel and very clean scent is I pour a couple of drops of vinegar in the bathwater and just soak in it. When you sit in the tub, the water will flush in and out of your vagina area, giving a nice cleanse. I also informed her to visit the health store where there are a variety of natural ways to cleanse the vagina.

She told me that she heard some of her friends mention a douche, but she was too embarrassed to ask them what a douche was used for. She explained to me that the country she is from does not really discuss things of that nature, so she has to gather information from the friends she is around with.

I told this young lady that she does not ever have to be embarrassed, and if it's anything she needs information on, I told her to come and sit down with me and I will tell her everything that I know about a woman's body.

I have an aunt that refuses to use over-the-counter products because she says they dry you out, and instead she uses organic products that contain teas and herbs. When I asked my aunt how does she like using organic products, she said she wishes every sister would use organic products.

This is why I stress the importance of informing your daughters to avoid them from asking someone else for information. Not only is it embarrassing for your daughter, but what does it say about you as a mother?

Suppositories

THE first time I found out about this product was from my mother. One day I saw her with the box, and I asked her what did she have in her hand and why was she using it. She explained to me that it was a product that women insert in their vaginas. My next question was why women insert this product into their vaginas; she said they use this product to clean out their vaginas and rid their vaginas of any bad odors. She pulled one of the suppositories out of the box and showed me. She took one out of the wrapper and showed me the proper steps to use it.

There are different kinds of suppositories. Some suppositories are scented, and then there are the unscented ones. What all young woman need to understand is that scented products could cause a yeast infection. Even though a large amount of my friends choose to cleanse their vaginas with these products, doctors tell us the vagina cleans itself naturally. How does an experienced woman handle a situation when a younger sister who is seeking answers approaches her? We inform them.

Sanitary Napkins

EACH month, a young woman will experience her menstrual cycle. When a woman has her menstrual cycle, she will need to purchase a box of napkins (pads). There are two kinds of sanitary napkins: there are the ones that are each individually wrapped and include sanitary wipes, then there are the ones that are just placed inside the box. There are also different sizes the sanitary napkin comes in. There are the long ones for overnight protection, and then there are the regular sizes. Each sanitary napkin will contain adhesive at the back of each pad. Remove the paper and place inside the seat of the panty.

Now that we have an understanding of what the sanitary napkin is used for, let's talk about the proper way of disposing the sanitary napkin. Below you will see I mentioned a few steps.

1. Remove the old sanitary napkin, clean with the wipes, and replace with the clean sanitary napkin.
2. Place the old sanitary napkin in the wrapper, or wrap some tissue around it and place in the garbage.

Do not do the following:

1. Flush the sanitary napkins down the toilet.
2. Place the sanitary napkin behind the toilet bowl on the floor.
3. Set the sanitary napkin on top of the disposal bin.

Panty Liners

WHAT is the purpose of a panty liner? The purpose of the panty liner is to avoid the panty seat from becoming moist from the woman's normal discharge. The reason why I choose to use the panty liner is that it provides a great level of comfort for me throughout the day. Some women choose not to wear panty liners for their own reasons, but I don't leave the house without wearing one.

Stories from Daughters

EACH story you are about to read is true, but the names have been changed to protect their identities.

Sha. I was able to sit down with a young woman by the name of Sha. I asked this young woman to relive the day that her mother spoke to her about the importance of hygiene. Sha responded by saying that day never existed. I must admit I was not surprised. We sat down for a moment, and she began to tell me a story about her menstrual cycle. Sha said she was about twelve years of age when she noticed blood in her pants. She explained to me that she was very scared because she did not know why she was bleeding. When she ran to her father and explained the situation to him, she said he immediately started to yell and scream at her. He called her mother and told her mother that she was having sex and she was pregnant. Her mother responded by saying she was not pregnant; she was just experiencing her menstrual cycle.

Sha was not only scared, but she was very confused. This is why mothers are supposed to inform their daughters about their bodies and what to expect at certain ages. The wrong way to inform your daughters is after things have presented themselves.

B. While I spoke to some women face-to-face, this conversation with B happened over the phone. I asked B a few questions about her sit-down talk with her mom.

She replied and told me that her mother never told her anything about hygiene. She said what she learned was not from her mother; it was from her aunt, and it was only bits and pieces of information. B explained to me that the man she was dating has a teenage daughter that comes over for the weekend, and this young woman does not know the importance of hygiene, and it's very clear that her mother is not taking the time out to teach her. B says every chance she gets, she takes the time out to tell her little things about her hygiene. B said she does not want to take the place of her mom, so she is very careful how she approaches and informs her stepdaughter.

These are necessary steps that B has taken. B clearly understands that she is not the mother of this young girl, but she is informing her about the proper way a young woman should take care of her body.

A. A is a young lady who I ride the train with some mornings. This is a young woman who was very open about her situations with her daughters. When I asked her about her approach to speaking to her daughters about their hygiene, she responded by saying it is a complicated situation because her daughter was raised by her mother for thirteen years. My next question was how she teaches her daughter about hygiene if her grandmother already taught her. A mentioned that she still talks to her daughter about cleaning after herself as she grows into a young woman. She mentioned her daughter does not really pay her any attention when she tries to talk to her about her hygiene, but as a mother, she has to continue to talk to her daughter.

How does a mother teach her daughter if someone else has already done so? What the mother has to do in a situation such as this one is learn what her daughter was taught and revise it. Teach your daughter, but most of all, watch her and see where her mistakes are being made.

I also informed A that regardless of the fact that the she did not raise her daughter from a child, she should not allow her daughter to use that against her, nor should she allow her daughter to make her feel guilty.

Ace. When I finally got the chance to sit down and speak to Ace, it was almost as if I opened Pandora's box. While Ace and I began to talk, her first response was "My mother never taught me anything about hygiene, and instead she degraded me by saying I would grow up to be a very bad mother." Ace said everything she ever learned about hygiene was from what she witnessed from being around her friends and aunts. This is a very hurtful situation. A mother's words should comfort and guide, not belittle and destroy. I asked Ace how she approaches her situation with her kids; she mentioned how she did the complete opposite of what her mother did to her. From the time they wake up in the morning down to the time they get ready for bed, she informs them of the importance of hygiene, and she encourages them in every direction they choose to take.

This situation could have turned out very different if Ace would have allowed her past to continue into her future, but instead she broke the cycle. Ace explained to me that children learn from their parents, and if their parents are not active in their daughter's life, then this allows someone else the opportunity to guide them. When a child is in the stages of growing, this is the time for mothers to talk to their daughters about hygiene. What I see all too often is parents trying to tell their daughters what to do after they're grown.

Barbara. I can remember an older woman who would come to me often for advice. Barbara had two daughters but was raising only one. I would often notice her youngest daughter did not pay that much of attention to her hygiene. She would come outside without brushing her teeth and she would have a body odor. I felt bad for this young girl because her mother was not teaching her the facts about life. This young girl would come outside, and she would be dressed as if she was living in the streets. She was fifteen years of age, and she was lost. I would give her clothing as well as coats and sneakers that I could not fit into anymore. I often thought to myself of the reason why her mother was not guiding her daughter, until one day she explained to me that her mother did not teach her anything about hygiene. After she confessed to me that her mother was not in her life, it all started to make sense. How does a parent teach her teenage daughter if her mother never taught her?

Throughout life, I often say to myself there is nothing wrong with not having an understanding, but there is definitely something wrong with not going to find help so that you may attain an understanding. The first time a mother smells her daughter, she is suppose to sit her down and explain to her daughter that young girls are never supposed to have a bad body odor. A mother is supposed to see as well as watch their daughters to make sure they're taking care of their bodies. Women that I spoke to said they learned on their own or someone else explained to them the importance of hygiene. It's sad and very touching because a large amount of these women learned the hard way. Kids are very mean, and being embarrassed is something you will never ever forget as a child.

Brit. Brit is a young woman who lives out of town with her boyfriend. When I had the chance to speak to Brit, she explained to me that her mother never sat her down and spoke to her about her hygiene. Brit said when she got her menstrual cycle, she called her mother at work and informed her mother that she was bleeding and did not know what to do about it. Brit said her mother told her to go to the store and get some maxi pads, pull the tape off, and put one on, and she will be fine. When I asked Brit how her mother talked to her about body odor, she said her mother never approached her, and she approached her mom instead. When Brit was a cheerleader, she said she began to notice that she had an underarm odor, so she went to her mother and said, "I think it's time that we go to the department store and purchase some deodorant." Her mother's response was "Girl, you don't need no deodorant. You are too young to wear deodorant." When I asked Brit how she learned the responsibilities as a young girl, she said she learned on her own.

When a daughter approaches her mother about a personal issue, this is the time for the mother to inform her daughter about everything she will experience as a growing young women. Even if a mother does not have the answers for her daughter's questions, then the mother needs to take the time and seek those answers, but mothers should never brush their daughters off.

Stages of Maturity

Relationships

BEFORE a relationship can prosper, the relationship should be evenly yoked, meaning the two individuals should believe in the same god. What I witnessed in relationships is when two people are going in the same direction and share the same dreams, they can relate to each other, and the relationships forms a tighter bond because of the similarities they share. When two people spend a large amount of time together, it allows the two to attain a greater understanding for each other, and the relationships forms a friendship bond also.

When a relationship begins, it is like watering a plant and watching it grow. If the plant is not watered and placed in sunlight, it will eventually wither away. The same effect takes place when a relationship does not contain love, respect, communication, and trust. When a relationship lacks these relevant words, the relationship fails.

When a woman begins a new relationship, the first thing she needs to understand is past relationships belong in the past. When a new relationship begins, it means a new start. Learn from your previous relationships and understand the reason for the breakup. Approach your current relationships with a new approach, and you will receive a different outcome.

Anytime a woman begins a new relationship, she needs to contain complete confidence in who she is. When a woman feels great about who she is, she will trust in her relationship and allow it to grow as opposed to not feeling great about herself and expecting a negative outcome.

I often hear women speaking about men and how all men are the same. the problem with this statement is they're all the same because you keep choosing the same type of man. If you're searching for a man who works on Wall Street, wears suits and ties, and eats at the finest restaurants, why are you in the clubs? The type of man you want to attract should coincide with the surroundings you attend.

Sisters, when you first meet a young man, from the very beginning of the conversation, the two of you should express what you expect in a relationship. Once this young man begins to tell you that he is not looking for a girl and he just wants to have fun, if this is not the direction you want to head in, then this would be the time to cease any further communication. What I witnessed from a large amount of sisters is you continue to see this man after you learned what he is about. You are hurting yourself. I must admit relationships are not easy, but they can be understood if you communicate with your mate.

Finance and a Relationship

Each woman I engage in a conversation with admits to wanting to live the life of the glitz and glamour. Please do not get me wrong; there is nothing wrong with wanting the best that life has to offer, but let me be the first to say you don't need a man to make those dreams become a reality.

Think about it, when you meet a man who drives a very expensive car, wears very expensive jewelry, lives in a huge home, and has a very successful business, what are the first words that come out your mouth when you mention this man to your girlfriends? Do you need help? You mention everything he owns. The key words to this conversation are he has. Yeah, you might get to ride in his car, visit his home and his business; he might even let you try on one of his chains, but guess what, when it's time for him to go home, everything you mentioned is going with him.

Let me explain the importance of you being a young, independent sister. You become your own woman, your direction is yours, you create your destiny, and you are in total control of your finance. When you allow a man to support you, he has total control over everything.

You create your bank account. You pay the rent on your apartment, and you buy the food and pay your own bills. You were born by yourself, so you are capable of taking care of yourself.

The best feeling I ever attained in life is taking care of me.

Good Relationships

A good relationship is one that brings complete happiness into the home as well as the heart. Couples are supposed to bring happiness into each other's life. When you love and care for a person, their interaction with the world should be a major concern. You want your partner to keep a smile on your face at all times. True lovebirds feel each other's pain. When a man loves a woman, he wants his woman looking and feeling her very best. A real man compliments his woman, and he makes her feel like a queen. A caring man will often tell his woman how beautiful she is, how he feels complete with her being in his life, and she is the best thing that has ever happened to him.

My young sisters, the type of men that you need in your life is the type of men that are going to guide you in the direction of success. My young sisters, you need to be with a man who offers his advice, but allows you to make your own decisions in life. A true man will tell you to complete school and attend college. A real man will offer his support and assist you in any way he can. A real man will be there when times are hard. A real man would never create stressful situations that would hurt you in the end.

It's very easy to know when you meet a man that wants to build you. He will often use the words like us and when, we, or my family. Men use words to express where your relationship stands.

Another way to tell that a man is very interested in you is he will want you to meet his mother as well as his family. His family will know of you before they even meet you.

For all my young sisters, you need to know that a real man will only bring you happiness.

Loyalty

Loyalty means a great deal in a relationship. Loyalty is the beginning of a great relationship. If you are in a relationship and cheating exists, the relationship will become complicated and very stressful. What I want each young sister to understand is that you will never be able to change a man; he has to be willing to change on his own. If you are dating a young man who has a problem being loyal to you, then you need to understand that he is not the man for you and you need to discontinue the relationship. Once a young man has cheated on you, he will most likely cheat again.

What I learned as a young girl maturing into a woman was a man can only do what we allow him to do. If a man wants to be with you, his actions will speak for itself. You will never ever have to ask questions like why did you not answer your phone? On the other hand, where were you? If a man loves you and wants to be with you, he is coming home to you.

Loyalty is the relationship, and without it, you have nothing.

Respect

Let me first inform you that respect starts with you respecting yourself. How can you expect others to respect you, and you are not respecting yourself?

Respect is not an action that takes place some of the time. Respect is a constant action that keeps repeating itself. Respect can be displayed in man's actions or a man's words.

If he doesn't respect his mother, why do you think he will respect you?

Encouragement

This is a very powerful word, and if it is used often, you can create an outstanding and very intelligent woman. Encouraging words are just the beginning to creating a very positive and outstanding young sister. As a mother, encourage your daughters to reach for their dreams. Inform them that there is no limit to what they can accomplish, and remember it is what you instill in them that creates who they become.

Bad Relationships

HE loves me. Or does he really? Let me tell you all about the bad relationships and the things they contain:

1. Dominance
2. Violence
3. Manipulation
4. Intimidation
5. Abuse – physically, emotionally, and mentally
6. Verbal abuse
7. Selfishness

These are just a few words to give you an example of the wrong men and their actions. Every word that I mentioned is just a few of the words that the wrong man will use.

A man who is against his woman will never support her, and his concern for her achieving great accomplishments will be limited. He will hold you back from your dreams and instead lead you into a path of complete destruction. Just think for a moment. Can you remember one time you where headed to school, but instead your boyfriend convinced you to play hooky? if you answered yes, then you know what type of man you're dealing with.

When you are in a relationship with a man who constantly breaks your spirit and tells you things like you are nothing and you will never be anything, then you know you are with a man whose purpose is destroying and controlling you.

Breaking your spirit, keeping you limited to only your current surroundings, moving you away and keeping you from your family, forcing you stay in the house and cater to his every need is what a selfish and sneaky man would do. Is he concerned for your safety? No, he wants to control you and destroy your every direction you attempt to take in life.

Self-esteem. The less you love yourself, the more you will allow and accept mistreatment and disrespect from others.

High Self-Esteem

This consists of an individual who has complete confidence in everything they attempt to achieve. They approach the most challenging and difficult situations with a conformation in advance. Morals, values, and standards are an interaction with their everyday existence. Unsure thoughts and doubt are excluded from their path in life. Elevation, excellence, and accomplishments are tools that will promote them to a level of prominence.

When a young woman has a high self-esteem level, she is equipped with a weapon that will allow her to reach for and achieve the best that life has to offer. Her level of confidence will not permit her to have thoughts of accepting anything less.

When a sister has a path and a plan, she has a life that will excel beyond her expectations. Self-esteem allows every aspect in a young woman's life to be meaningful.

Our daughters' self-esteem is formed by the words we instill in them. Encourage your daughters to reach for their dream no matter how impossible it may sound.

Let me tell you a fact. Young sisters who are raised from birth to love themselves, take care of their appearance, set goals, and believe in their dreams are young woman who grow up to become great lawyers, excellent doctors, architects, judges, etc. As long as your daughters continuously hear the words yes, you can, than yes, she will.

Low Self-Esteem

This consists of doubt, neglect, fear, and abuse. When women are dealing with low self-esteem, it will not be complicated to detect. What I noticed from young women who have low self-esteem is they will tend to neglect their appearance, accept disrespect in their relationships, contain no motivation, and they will settle for less.

Low self-esteem keeps young sisters afraid as well as content with their surroundings. They're afraid to reach for change for fear of failure because their entire life was complete with words that destroyed and damaged their chance to begin to dream.

Dreams of attending college and becoming your own boss are nowhere in the thought process. Succeeding in life and becoming a prominent figure in society does not exist. Becoming the first female president is impossible. Their thoughts are limited to their surroundings. Everything that happens to their life that's negative is what they deserve. So they believe.

It is very sad to mention these statements, but unfortunately, these are the dreams of young women who have no self-esteem.

When young women are being abused in the streets, or when we see young women who are being sold by pimps and trained by prostitutes, it's because this is all they think they are worth. Low self-esteem is weakening, it's degrading, and it's almost impossible to think you can do better.

A caring man will build you; an evil man will destroy you.

Rape

IF your mother never told you, rape is the worst crime a person can commit. I don't care how old you are; you can go home and tell your mother what happened to you. Even if he tells you what he will do to you if you ever tell. If you don't tell your mother what happened to you, he will do it again.

Anytime you tell a man no and he still climbs on top of you and injects himself inside of you, then that is considered rape. Anytime a man touches your body and you tell him to stop and he continues, this is a crime. What I want you to remember is no man has the right to force you to do anything against your will, and anytime you find yourself in a situation like this, you tell everybody. Never keep that a secret.

Men who rape women will be placed in prison for many years, but the only way he will stop raping you is if you tell what he has done to you. I do not care who the man is – your father, your uncle, your brother, or your cousin. It does not make it right. According to RAINN (Rape, Abuse, and Incest National Network), "44% of victims are under 18, 80% are under 30, every 107 seconds, another American is sexually assaulted. Each year there are about 293,000 victims of sexual assault. 68% of assaults are not reported to police. 98% of rapists will never spend time a day in jail or prison."

Date Rape

Sisters, when you young women meet men on the Internet dating network, before you even think of going on a date with this person, you should get to know what he is about. There are so many men in the Internet whose main purpose is to lure young women in and take advantage of them.

When you go on a date with a man, the first thing you should do is not accept any forms of alcohol from this man. Date rape occurs often. When you accept a drink of any kind from a man, you are putting yourself at risk for rape.

When your drink is left unattended and you walk away from it, once you return, throw the drink in the garbage. Pay attention to men who are persistent to buy you drinks. You will not know if a pill has been dropped into your drink until it is too late. Pay attention when you are out on a date.

Pregnancy

WHEN young women begin to have intercourse with their boyfriends, there are many risks. First, let me begin by saying there is plenty of time to start planning to have a baby after you achieved your high school diploma and graduated from college. Some young girls feel as though having a baby is cool because all their friends are having babies, but the fact is having a baby can put your life on hold.

My young sisters, it is not easy raising children when your education is limited and your financial situation depends on the public assistance program. It is sad because my young sisters are having babies for all the wrong reasons. I have heard young girls often say "I'm going to have his baby because he has good hair and he is cute." I have also heard young girls often say "My baby is going to be dressed with all the latest brand-name clothes."

Raising a child is not an easy step. When a baby is born, the mother will have to wake up in the middle of the night and feed the baby, check the baby's Pampers to see if the baby is wet, burp the baby, and then rock the baby back to sleep. All babies need clean clothes and a warm home. Babies have to take baths, and their skin has to be taken care of. Babies have to go to the doctors for their immunizations shots. A baby needs clothes, shoes, and Pampers. There are programs that supply mothers with WIC checks, but what happens when the WIC checks run out? You will have to buy the milk with your funds until the next WIC pickup date. It is not about dressing your baby in all the flashiest cloths, but it is about taking the time to care for your baby as well as spending time with your child.

Just let me tell all my young sisters this: once your baby is born, it is not about you anymore; it is about that baby and supplying the baby with all the basic needs. All those brand-name jeans, coats, shoes, and jewelry that you used to wear will no longer exist because your child has to be taken care of now. All the parties and staying out late in the clubs will come to an end, and you will have to be home to take care of that child that you gave birth to.

Sister, please disregard when a man tells you that he will be there to help you take care of the child or he will help watch the baby. This sounds great, but to be honest, whether he chooses to be there or not, you as a mother have no choice but to take care and provide for that baby. According to CDC (Centers for Disease Control and Prevention), "In 2012, a total of 305,388 babies were born to women ages 15–19 years, for a live birth rate of 29.4 per 1,000 women in this age group."

Abortions

ABORTION should not be used as a form of birth control. Abortions not only kill growing babies, but also the continuous scraping destroys the female walls, causing severe damage to your stomach lining.

I heard many conversations where young women talk about getting abortions like it so simple. There are so many women that cannot have children because of their actions as a young girl. Abortions not only kill a growing fetus, but the mother who is having the procedure is also in great danger.

Each time a woman goes to have an abortion, she is being damaged mentally as well as physically. There are so many risks when having an abortion.

1. Hemorrhaging can accrue.
2. Breathing difficulties can accrue.
3. The baby can be lodged in a woman's tubes, which can not only be very dangerous, but can cause extreme pain.
4. There can be side effects from the medication that is administrated while the procedure is taking place.

There was this one sister whom I would give advice to concerning her boyfriend. One day she came to me and told me she was pregnant, but her boyfriend did not want her to have this baby. She started crying and then she started confessing to me how he also cheats on her and abuses her. So I asked her two questions: The first one was why does she stay with him. The second question was what she was going to do about the baby that was growing inside her stomach.

Her first response to the first question was "I love him." The second answer was she had no idea what she was going to do about the baby. What I told her to do was go and tell her mother that she was pregnant. After about a week, I saw her again, and she told me she had an abortion. She also told me she was still with him. After about a month, I saw her again, and she said she was pregnant again and she was going to have another abortion. I was very disturbed because I felt like the first time she confessed to her mother, there should have been some type of action taken so that she would not have to go through this same situation again.

I went home and I sat down and thought about her, and I tried my best to figure out what type of advice her mother gave her, because she was going to have her second abortion. What her mother should have done was take her to the doctor's office so that she could be placed on birth control. It was too late to stop her from having sex, but it was not too late to prevent her from getting pregnant again. According to Choices Pregnancy Care Center, "There were an estimated 1.21 million abortions in the U.S. in 2008 (3,322 abortions per day). 17% of all U.S. abortions are from teenagers."

The Welfare System

I WANT to give a brief breakdown on why the welfare system was created. Welfare was created in 1930 by local and state governments/private charities. What prompted the government to take action was the fact that men, women, and children were starving because of the Great Depression that was caused by the stock market collapse in 1929.

This system (the New Deal) was created by President Franklin D. Roosevelt to help families financially with the basic means to survive. This system went through different stages from the year 1929 until today, 2015.

These rules changed drastically in the year 1996, when President Bill Clinton created the Personal Responsibility and Work Opportunity Reconciliation Act (PRWORA). This system was signed into law by President Bill Clinton on August 22, 1996.

According to TeenHelp.com, "80 percent of unmarried teen mothers end up on Welfare."

According to the U.S. Census Bureau, "out of about 12 million single parent families in 2014 more than 80% were headed by single mothers. Today 1 in 4 children under the age of 18–a total of about 17.4 million are being raised without a father and nearly half (45%) live below the poverty line."

A Baby Will Not Keep Him

MANY young girls believe that once they have a baby with a man, he will stay with them. It is very sad because most of the time the man feels like he is being trapped because the woman wants to have his baby, so instead of staying with the woman, he leaves her and the baby.

If a man tells you he does not want to have a baby, then why do you even allow him to get you pregnant? My young sisters, you are responsible for your acts, and if you know he does not want any kids, you have three choices: use condoms, go to the doctor's and get some birth control pills, or refrain from having sex until you get married. A responsible man will take the necessary steps to avoid an unwanted pregnancy. An irresponsible man will create an unwanted pregnancy and then abandon it.

Having a baby should be an exciting moment. Why would you have a baby and you have to chase down the young man who got you pregnant so he can help you take care of this baby? My young sisters, every time you think about having a baby, I want you to pay attention to your friends struggling with raising a child as a single parent, and I want you to wait before you make that same mistake. According to teen sex and pregnancy. Facts in brief. AGI. 1999 "each year 10% of all women aged 15–19 become pregnant. Every year 1 in 5 women aged 15–19 who had sex become pregnant. 78% of teen pregnancies are unintended."

Diseases

THIS topic is dangerous. If your mother never told you, protection is needed often. To all my young sisters who are unaware of the deadly diseases that exist in today's society, there are many. I just mentioned a few that has a very high rate in today's society.

These diseases have affected a large amount of my family and friends, and they continue to destroy many lives by the day. These diseases can touch the lives of everyone, and just for your information, they do not discriminate.

1. AIDS
2. Chlamydia
3. Scabies
4. Syphilis
5. Herpes

What is scary about contracting these diseases is the individual's motives. People who have them will not inform you that they're infected. They will purposely infect others because someone infected them.

Each one of the diseases that I mentioned has different symptoms, causes, as well as effects that can damage or destroy the entire immune system.

A person who is suffering from a sickness will not wear it stamped on their foreheads, nor will they inform you in advance of their sickness. This is a society that's filled with evil people who want company in their unfortunate situation. According to the American Sexual Health Association, "recent estimates from the Centers for Disease Control and Prevention show that there are 19.7 million new STI every year in the U.S. In 2008, there were an estimated 110 million prevalent STI among women and men in the U.S. Of these, more than 20% (22.1 million) were among women and men aged 15 to 24 years. Each year, one in four teens contract an STD/STI."

Pap Test

IF your mother never told you, it is very important that woman visit their doctor often. Every woman's body is different and can experience a variety of complications. That is why it is very important that young women take the necessary steps to take care of their health by visiting the doctor's and keeping their doctor's appointments. A woman needs to take a Pap smear test at least every six months out of the year. This test is very important because it detects any signs of infections that can be life threatening. Infections that could be life threatening. According to the American Academy of Family Physicians, "ages 21 to 30, you should have a pap test every three years."

Early prevention is always the best.

Gynecology

Every young woman must visit the doctor at least every six months. This doctor deals with a woman's vaginal area. When you visit this doctor, tests will be completed, and for any signs of abnormities you will be notified. The purpose for this doctor is to treat, destroy, and prevent any signs of growth inside of the woman's body. This doctor is very important, and every young sister needs to visit one. The American College of Obstetricians and Gynecologist (ACOG) recommends that girls should first see a gynecologist when they are between the ages of thirteen and fifteen.

Take care of yourself.

Drugs

THIS topic is a topic that destroys young sisters by the dozen. There are large amounts of drugs that have hit the streets. These drugs are being mixed with all forms of different ingredients. Here is a story I want to speak about to show my young sisters how drugs can destroy your life and cause you to lose everything you worked so hard for.

The reason I chose to speak about drugs is that I have seen so many young women hooked on drugs and turn tricks to support their drug habit. I can remember attending junior high school; there was a girl that always came to school looking great. Her hair was always done, and her clothes were always nice and neat. Years later and on occasions, I see this same girl, and she looks terrible. She is doing drugs, and she even looks like she may be homeless and sleeping on the streets. Every time I see her, I want to stop her and ask her what happened and were did she go wrong in life. How does someone go from looking and doing great in society to being a drug user and destroying her life? Many times, young women begin using drugs because of pressure from their friends. When kids start using drugs to please their friends, it's because they want to fit in and be cool. It is very sad because if a mother does not inform their daughters about the dangers when using drugs, they will fall victim to the drug dealers.

I have seen a beautiful young woman at the tender age of fifteen become involved with an older man who was thirty years of age, and he turned her completely out. If her mother would have warned her about drugs and walking away when someone offers her drugs, she would have been prepared to deal with this situation. She went from smoking crack to turning tricks. Every time I would see this young woman, she would have a black eye, and her facial expressions were often sad. I had the opportunity to speak to this young sister one day, and I asked her why she stays with a man who abuses her. She said if she left him, he would find her, beat her up, and force her to return home with him.

I asked this young sister many questions. My first question was where was her mother and if her mother was alive. My next question was if she had any family members who could help her get away from this man. She said yes, she has family who cares about her and wants her to come home, but her decision was to stay with this man.

The information I found out just through hearing conversations in the street was this older man was her pimp. He controlled her life, destroyed her self-esteem, and convinced her no one will ever want her. She lived in complete darkness and fear. Even if this mother was able to convince her daughter to leave this man, the damage has already been done; he broke her spirit and destroyed her to the point where she felt worthless, useless, and dirty.

This is only one in a million stories of young women who have been abused, hooked on drugs, and forced to prostitute. This is the reason why I wrote this book to inform my young sisters the dangers they will face in the streets.

My young sisters, please understand once you begin to use drugs, your life will be destroyed and your body will deteriorate. Remember what I told you and keep it with you for a lifetime, and anytime you are unsure and need guidance, pray to God, and he will guide you in the correct direction.

Nothing good will ever come from using drugs. According to Project Know, understanding addiction "CBS News reports that a recent survey indicates approximately two million teens between the ages of 12 and 17 currently need treatment for substance abuse problem, but only about 150,000 get the help they need."

The Correct Order to Attain an Excellent Life

1. Complete public school.
2. Complete junior high school and high school.
3. Attend college.
4. Get your associate's degree.
5. Get your bachelor's degree.
6. Get your master's degree.
7. And then attain your doctorate.
8. Start your career.
9. Maintain good credit.
10. Buy a house/condo.
11. Purchase your dream car.
12. Start dating.
13. Get into a relationship.
14. Get married.
15. Have kids.

It touches me when so many of our young daughters go through life in the wrong order. There are steps to climbing the ladder of success, but not everyone will follow them. Unfortunately, I was one of those young women who followed these steps, but in the incorrect order.

When you complete public school, you take what you learned in public school and apply it to your subjects in junior high school. Once you graduate from junior high school, you take your lessons from junior high school and apply them to high school. There are orders as well as levels that must be taken before you can proceed to the advanced stages, which would be your college years.

I will not tell you that it's too late to return and complete school, but I will tell you when you step outside of the correct orders, you will definitely have a complicated road to travel.

I had two sons out of wedlock, I did not complete high school when I was supposed to, I received public assistance, and everything about relationships I had to learn the hard way. Yeah, my mother told me some things, but everything she did not tell me caused me to travel through life of struggle and pain! Information is relevant.

The older I become, the more I understand that there are two ways to travel through life: there is the right way, and then there is the wrong way. The right way allows you to become a very successful young woman who achieves all her goals, graduates with honors, and is optimistic for her future. Approaching life the wrong way by procrastinating and making up excuses as to why you cannot achieve your goal will definitely keep you stagnated.

Learn from this information that you have just read, understand that there are two ways to travel through life to reach your goals, and allow your dreams to come true through hope, faith, and perseverance.

There's a reason why everything has order.

Whatever Happened to Parents Introducing Their Daughters to School Activities?

MOMS, there are so many activities that are free of charge. What I noticed about young sisters who are active are that they are less likely to go astray. Every school system has a variety of activities; inform and encourage your daughters to participate.

Learn what excites your daughter, and encourage her to create and introduce her dream as an activity. If she is interested in the cheerleader team, she might want to create their uniforms, or what about creating plays by using her friends' personal experiences? There is the basketball team, volleyball team, dance class, arts and crafts. A child should never ever say they're bored.

If your daughter has a desire to bring something to life, you as her mother must assist and support her. Whatever it is she wishes to do in life, you make it your business to place her in that area. Every day that passes, make sure she works on her project until she brings that dream to life.

Inform her of starting her own business and being her own boss. What I'm trying to get you as parents to understand is the more young women are kept busy, the less they will become involved with those who are heading in the wrong direction.

Rewarding Your Daughter for Her Accomplishments

Every time your daughter's school grades are in great standards, she should be rewarded. Let her know that you recognize her great accomplishments and you believe in her. The more you reward her for the small accomplishments, the more she will proceed to the great accomplishments. Surprise her with tickets to see a Broadway play, or purchase a tennis bracelet. Purchase her favorite lotion scent and place it on her bed with a nice card so that she is surprised when she gets home from school. It is very important that your daughter knows that she is heading in the correct direction and her mother recognizes her accomplishments.

Punishing Your Daughter for Unacceptable Behavior

When your daughter oversteps her boundaries, your daughter needs to be punished if her grades have fallen below excellence. Show her that the grades she is bringing home are not acceptable and explain to her that her current grades are a reflection of what she is not doing in class.

Never reward a daughter when she is not doing great things. If you reward a child when she is doing bad things, she will think it's okay and she will continue to go astray. You do not have to confine your daughter to the home, but when she is not doing what you expect her to do, then punish her and remove her favorite things from her grasp.

Restrict her from watching TV, temporarily remove her cell phone, and minimize all contact from her friends after school hours. During the weekends, she should not be allowed to go outside for anything, and make her go to bed extra early, but you cannot feel sorry for your daughter because she looks sad and she is crying. Stick to this punishment and show her that you mean business, and she will not neglect her school assignments anymore.

Throughout the pages of this book are lessons that I also encountered as a young sister maturing into a woman. Life has many lessons to be learned, but my reason for informing my young sisters is hopes that they will learn before experiencing the hardships that come along with life.

I want each one of my young sisters to have the chance to achieve before failure. I created this book in hopes that my young sisters will learn and refrain from their current direction. They need to understand that there is so much more in life than what they are reaching and settling for.

Conclusion

THROUGHOUT the pages of this book, you will notice how my life went from adversity to triumphs. The entire reason for producing this book was to offer information, submit my personal experiences, and divert my young sisters attention from being content with their current situation to comprehending that there is an entire world of opportunity. I pray that the words touched each and every young sister that took the time to read this book. In addition, I hope this book clarified the misconceptions of a young woman's presentation of herself and allowed her to recreate her current situation.

Acknowledgement

To my mom who did her best in raising and guiding me,
I pray you are resting in peace.

To my dad, love and miss you. I know you are close to me daily.

To my sons, Mike and Si, I love you and thank God for you.

To My Heart, my friend, and my protector, Dee, you are amazing.
Words can't describe the man you are. I feel you in my soul. I love you, Mister.

To my only sister, Dawn (Maria), you are my best friend. I adore you. Muah.

To my brother-in-law, Stanley, your favorite words are "God is good." I must
agree–yes, he is. Thank you for your Bible classes.

To my brothers, Mike and Roy, I love you, guys.

To my uncle Jay, you should have been the president.

www.ingramcontent.com/pod-product-compliance
Lightning Source LLC
Chambersburg PA
CBHW050340290526
45785CB00006B/2572